THE OSTEOPOROSIS DIET

A Comprehensive Guide to Eating for Strong Bones

COPYRIGHT © 2023

All rights reserved.

No part of this book may be reproduced in any form or by any electronic or mechanical means, including information storage and retrieval systems, without permission in writing from the publisher, except by a reviewer who may quote brief passages in a review.

The information contained in this book is based on the author's research and experience. While the author has made every effort to provide accurate and up-to-date information, errors and omissions may occur. The author and publisher assume no responsibility for any errors or omissions or for any actions taken based on the information contained in this book.

The information contained in this book is provided "as is," without warranty of any kind, express or implied, including but not limited to the warranties of merchantability, fitness for a particular purpose, or non-infringement. In no event shall the author or publisher be liable for any claim, damages, or other liability, whether in an action of contract, tort, or otherwise, arising from, out of, or in connection with the book or the use or other dealings in the book.

TABLE OF CONTENTS

INTRODUCTION

Osteoporosis is a common and debilitating medical condition that affects the skeletal system, leading to weakened bones and an increased risk of fractures. This silent and often asymptomatic disease is characterized by a reduction in bone density and the deterioration of bone tissue, resulting in bones becoming fragile and susceptible to fractures even with minimal trauma or stress. Osteoporosis primarily affects older adults, particularly postmenopausal women, although it can occur in men as well. It is a significant global health concern, with far-reaching implications for individuals' quality of life, healthcare systems, and public health efforts. Understanding the causes, risk factors, prevention strategies, and management of osteoporosis is vital in addressing this pervasive and potentially debilitating condition.

Osteoporosis, a prevalent and debilitating medical condition, represents a significant public health challenge worldwide. The hallmark feature of osteoporosis is the progressive deterioration of bone tissue, which renders bones fragile and prone to fractures, even with minimal trauma or stress. What makes this condition particularly insidious is that it often advances silently over many years, often without noticeable symptoms until a fracture occurs. These fractures can have severe consequences, leading to chronic pain, disability, reduced quality of life, and increased healthcare costs.

Osteoporosis is influenced by various factors, including genetics, hormonal changes (especially in postmenopausal women), aging, lifestyle choices, and nutrition. As such, prevention, early detection, and management strategies are of paramount importance. Individuals at risk of osteoporosis are encouraged to adopt a multifaceted approach to their health, encompassing lifestyle modifications, dietary adjustments, weight-bearing exercises, and, in some cases, medications prescribed by healthcare professionals.

This introduction aims to provide an overview of the complex nature of osteoporosis, shedding light on its underlying causes, risk factors, health impact, and the importance of early intervention. By understanding the intricate interplay of factors involved in this condition and the significance of proactive measures, individuals can take proactive steps to mitigate the impact of osteoporosis on their lives and maintain strong and resilient bones throughout their lifespan.

An osteoporosis diet, also known as a bone-healthy diet, plays a pivotal role in the prevention and management of osteoporosis, a condition characterized by weakened bones with reduced bone density and increased susceptibility to fractures. This dietary approach is centered around optimizing nutrient intake to support bone health, enhance bone density, and minimize the risk of fractures. A well-balanced osteoporosis diet emphasizes specific nutrients like calcium, vitamin D, magnesium, and protein, while also focusing on maintaining a healthy body weight and reducing the consumption of substances that can negatively impact bone health, such as excessive sodium and caffeine. In this comprehensive dietary plan, individuals are encouraged to include foods rich in these essential nutrients, engage in weight-bearing exercises, and adopt a holistic approach to overall wellness to minimize the impact of osteoporosis on their quality of life and physical well-being. This introduction will delve deeper into the key elements of an osteoporosis diet, providing insight into the importance of each dietary component and how they collectively contribute to the promotion of strong and resilient bones.

PART ONE

WHAT IS OSTEOPOROSIS?

Osteoporosis is a medical condition characterized by the weakening of bones, which leads to a decrease in bone density and an increased risk of fractures. It is often referred to as a "silent disease" because it typically progresses without noticeable symptoms until a fracture occurs. Osteoporosis causes bones to become fragile and porous, making them more susceptible to fractures, even with minor stresses or falls that would not normally cause a fracture in healthy bones.

SYMPTOMS

Osteoporosis is often referred to as a "silent disease" because it typically progresses without noticeable symptoms until a fracture occurs. Many individuals with osteoporosis may not be aware that they have the condition until they experience a fracture or have a bone density test. However, in some cases, especially as osteoporosis progresses, individuals may experience certain symptoms and signs, including:

• Bone Pain: Some people with osteoporosis may develop bone pain, particularly in the spine or other areas where fractures have occurred. This pain can be chronic and may worsen with physical activity or when lifting objects.

• Loss of Height: Vertebral fractures (fractures in the spine) can lead to a loss of height over time and may result in a stooped or hunched posture (kyphosis). This change in posture is sometimes referred to as a "dowager's hump."

• Change in Body Shape: As the spine becomes more curved due to vertebral fractures, there may be a noticeable change in the overall shape of the body.

• Frequent Fractures: Individuals with advanced osteoporosis may experience fractures more easily than expected, even with minor trauma or falls.

It's important to note that these symptoms are typically associated with the consequences of osteoporosis, such as fractures, rather than the condition itself. Therefore, the absence of symptoms does not necessarily mean an absence of osteoporosis.

To detect and diagnose osteoporosis before fractures occur, healthcare providers often recommend bone density testing, such as a dual-energy X-ray absorptiometry (DXA) scan. These tests can identify reduced bone density and the risk of fractures, allowing for early intervention and management to prevent further bone loss and fractures. If you have concerns about your bone health or risk factors for osteoporosis, it's important to discuss them with your healthcare provider.

RISK FACTORS AND HOW TO IDENTIFY THEM

Identifying risk factors for osteoporosis is crucial for early detection, prevention, and management of the condition. Here are some common risk factors and how to identify them:

• Age: The risk of osteoporosis increases with age, especially for women. Postmenopausal women are at a higher risk due to hormonal changes. Men also face an increased risk as they age.

• Gender: Women are more likely to develop osteoporosis than men. This is primarily due to the decrease in estrogen levels during menopause, which accelerates bone loss.

• Family History: A family history of osteoporosis or fractures can increase your risk. If your parents or siblings have had osteoporosis or fractures, you may be at a higher risk.

• Menopause: For women, early onset of menopause (before age 45) or surgical removal of the ovaries can increase the risk of osteoporosis due to a rapid decline in estrogen levels.

• Low Body Weight: Being underweight or having a low body mass index (BMI) can increase the risk of osteoporosis, as there is less bone mass to begin with.

• Hormone Levels: Hormonal imbalances, such as low estrogen in women and low testosterone in men, can contribute to bone loss. Identifying hormonal issues may require blood tests conducted by a healthcare provider.

• Dietary Factors: A diet low in calcium and vitamin D can increase the risk of osteoporosis. If your diet lacks these nutrients or if you have malabsorption issues, you may be at risk.

• Physical Activity: A sedentary lifestyle or lack of weight-bearing exercise can contribute to bone loss. Identifying low levels of physical activity can be done through self-assessment or consultation with a healthcare provider.

• Smoking: Smoking is a risk factor for osteoporosis. If you smoke or have a history of smoking, this can increase your risk.

• Excessive Alcohol Consumption: Consuming more than two alcoholic drinks per day for women and more than three for men can contribute to bone loss.

• Certain Medications: Long-term use of medications such as corticosteroids (e.g., prednisone) can weaken bones. If you are on such medications, your healthcare provider should monitor your bone health.

• Medical Conditions: Certain medical conditions, including celiac disease, Crohn's disease, rheumatoid arthritis, and hormonal disorders, can increase the risk of osteoporosis.

• Previous Fractures: If you've had a previous fracture as an adult, especially from a minor fall or impact, it may be an indicator of underlying osteoporosis.

To identify these risk factors, consider the following steps:

• Review your personal and family medical history.

• Assess your lifestyle and dietary habits.

• Discuss your concerns and risk factors with a healthcare provider, who can perform necessary tests and evaluations.

• Bone density testing, such as a DXA scan, is a key diagnostic tool that can assess bone health and fracture risk. Your healthcare provider can recommend this test if deemed necessary based on your risk factors.

Identifying and understanding your risk factors is the first step in managing and reducing your risk of osteoporosis through lifestyle changes, dietary adjustments, and medical interventions when necessary. Regular discussions with a healthcare provider are essential to monitor bone health and take appropriate preventive measures.

DIAGNOSIS

The diagnosis of osteoporosis typically involves a combination of clinical evaluation, medical history assessment, and bone density testing. Here are the key steps involved in diagnosing osteoporosis:

• Medical History and Risk Assessment: Your healthcare provider will begin by taking a detailed medical history. They will ask about your family history of osteoporosis, any previous fractures, menopausal status (for women), lifestyle factors such as diet, physical activity, smoking, and alcohol consumption, and any underlying medical conditions or medications that may affect bone health.

• Physical Examination: A physical examination may be conducted to assess for signs of osteoporosis-related changes, such as loss of height, stooped posture, and spinal deformities. This can help identify any physical symptoms or manifestations of the condition.

• Bone Density Testing: The most common and definitive way to diagnose osteoporosis is through bone density testing. The gold standard for measuring bone density is a dual-energy X-ray absorptiometry (DXA) scan. This non-invasive test measures bone mineral density (BMD) in the hip, spine, or wrist. It provides a T-score, which compares your BMD to that of a healthy young adult of the same gender. The results are used to classify bone health as follows:

a. Normal: T-score above -1

b. Osteopenia (low bone mass): T-score between -1 and -2.5

c. Osteoporosis: T-score at or below -2.5

• Laboratory Tests: Blood tests may be conducted to assess hormonal levels (such as estrogen and testosterone) and to rule out underlying medical conditions that could contribute to bone loss.

• Fracture Assessment: If you've had a fracture as an adult, especially a fragility fracture (one that occurs with minimal or no trauma), your healthcare provider may consider this as an indication of underlying osteoporosis.

• Additional Imaging: In some cases, additional imaging studies like vertebral fracture assessments (VFA) or X-rays of the spine may be performed to detect vertebral fractures that are not apparent on clinical examination.

• Evaluation of Other Risk Factors: Your healthcare provider will consider other risk factors for osteoporosis, such as family history, lifestyle factors, and medications, in conjunction with bone density testing to make a comprehensive diagnosis.

Once a diagnosis of osteoporosis or osteopenia is confirmed, your healthcare provider will discuss treatment and management options. These may include lifestyle modifications (such as diet and exercise), medications to strengthen bones, and regular monitoring of bone health.

It's important to note that early detection and diagnosis of osteoporosis are essential for timely intervention and the prevention of fractures. If you have concerns about your bone health or risk factors for osteoporosis, it's crucial to discuss them with a healthcare provider, who can assess your individual risk, recommend appropriate testing, and develop a personalized plan to manage and mitigate the impact of the condition.

The treatment of osteoporosis aims to strengthen bones, reduce the risk of fractures, and manage the underlying condition. Treatment options for osteoporosis include lifestyle changes, dietary adjustments, medications, and other supportive measures. The choice of treatment depends on the severity of the condition, individual risk factors, and the recommendations of a healthcare provider. Here are some common treatment options:

1. Lifestyle Modifications:

• Diet: Ensure an adequate intake of calcium and vitamin D through a balanced diet. Include foods rich in these nutrients, or consider supplements if dietary intake is insufficient.

• Weight-Bearing Exercise: Engage in regular weight-bearing exercises such as walking, jogging, dancing, and strength training. These activities help stimulate bone growth and maintain bone density.

• Smoking Cessation: Quit smoking, as smoking can weaken bones and interfere with bone healing.

• Moderate Alcohol Consumption: Limit alcohol intake to moderate levels, as excessive alcohol consumption can negatively impact bone health.

2. Medications:

• Bisphosphonates: These are a class of medications that slow down bone loss and reduce the risk of fractures. Examples include alendronate (Fosamax), risedronate (Actonel), and zoledronic acid (Reclast).

• Hormone Replacement Therapy (HRT): In some cases, postmenopausal women may consider HRT to increase estrogen levels and slow bone loss. This option should be discussed with a healthcare provider, considering the potential risks and benefits.

• Selective Estrogen Receptor Modulators (SERMs): Medications like raloxifene (Evista) can mimic the positive effects of estrogen on bone health without affecting other tissues.

• Denosumab: This medication (Prolia) is an antibody that blocks a molecule involved in bone breakdown. It is administered by injection every six months.

• Parathyroid Hormone (Teriparatide): Teriparatide (Forteo) is a synthetic form of parathyroid hormone that can stimulate bone formation and is used in specific cases.

3. Calcium and Vitamin D Supplements:

For individuals who cannot get enough calcium and vitamin D through diet, supplements may be recommended. The dosage should be tailored to individual needs and often guided by blood test results.

4. Fall Prevention:

Implement strategies to prevent falls, such as removing tripping hazards at home, ensuring proper lighting, and using assistive devices as needed.

5. Fracture Management:

If a fracture occurs, prompt and appropriate medical care is crucial. This may involve pain management, immobilization, and rehabilitation.

6. Regular Monitoring:

Individuals with osteoporosis should have regular follow-up appointments with their healthcare provider to assess bone density, evaluate treatment efficacy, and adjust treatment plans as needed.

It's important to note that the choice of treatment should be individualized based on a person's risk factors, overall health, and preferences. Healthcare providers will work with individuals to develop a treatment plan that aligns with their specific needs and goals.

Additionally, osteoporosis treatment is often a long-term commitment, and adherence to the prescribed regimen is crucial for its effectiveness. Regular communication with a healthcare provider and adherence to the recommended treatment plan are essential for managing osteoporosis and reducing the risk of fractures.

BENEFITS AND POTENTIAL SIDE EFFECTS OF EACH TREATMENT OPTIONS

Each treatment option for osteoporosis comes with its own set of benefits and potential side effects. The choice of treatment should be based on individual factors, including the severity of the condition, underlying health concerns, and the recommendations of a healthcare provider. Here's an overview of the benefits and potential side effects of common osteoporosis treatments:

1. Lifestyle Modifications:

Benefits:

• Improves overall bone health.

• Supports general well-being.

• Low or no risk of side effects.

Potential Side Effects:

• None associated with adopting a healthy lifestyle.

• Adherence to dietary and exercise changes may be challenging for some individuals.

2. Calcium and Vitamin D Supplements:

Benefits:

• Ensures adequate intake of essential bone-strengthening nutrients.

• May reduce the risk of fractures when dietary intake is insufficient.

Potential Side Effects:

• Generally considered safe when taken as directed.

• Excessive intake can lead to side effects such as kidney stones or constipation.

3. Medications:

a. Bisphosphonates (e.g., alendronate, risedronate, zoledronic acid):

Benefits:

• Slows down bone loss and reduces fracture risk.

• May increase bone density.

Potential Side Effects:

• Gastrointestinal side effects, including heartburn, nausea, and stomach pain.

• Rarely, more serious side effects like osteonecrosis of the jaw and atypical femoral fractures, although these are very rare.

b. Hormone Replacement Therapy (HRT):

Benefits:

• Can increase bone density.

• May relieve menopausal symptoms.

Potential Side Effects:

• Increased risk of blood clots, breast cancer, and heart disease.

• Should be used with caution, and the decision should be based on individual risks and benefits.

c. Selective Estrogen Receptor Modulators (SERMs) (e.g., raloxifene):

Benefits:

• Can reduce the risk of spine fractures.

• No increased risk of breast cancer.

Potential Side Effects:

• Hot flashes, leg cramps, and an increased risk of blood clots (similar to HRT).

d. Denosumab:

Benefits:

• Slows down bone loss and reduces fracture risk.

Potential Side Effects:

• Increased risk of infections, including serious skin and bone infections.

• Hypocalcemia (low calcium levels).

• Possible association with atypical femoral fractures and osteonecrosis of the jaw.

e. Parathyroid Hormone (Teriparatide):

Benefits:

• Stimulates bone formation and increases bone density.

Potential Side Effects:

• May cause nausea, dizziness, and leg cramps.

• Limited to a two-year course of treatment.

It's important to discuss the benefits and potential side effects of each treatment option with a healthcare provider. The choice of treatment should be based on an individual's specific needs and risk factors. Regular follow-up with a healthcare provider is also crucial to monitor treatment effectiveness and adjust the treatment plan as necessary. Additionally, individuals should report any unusual or severe side effects promptly to their healthcare provider.

IMPORTANCE OF EARLY DETECTION

Early detection of osteoporosis is of paramount importance for several critical reasons:

• Prevention of Fractures: Osteoporosis is often referred to as a "silent disease" because it progresses silently, typically without symptoms, until a fracture occurs. By identifying the condition early, healthcare providers can intervene with preventive measures and treatments to reduce the risk of fractures. Fractures associated with osteoporosis can have severe consequences, leading to chronic pain, disability, and a reduced quality of life.

• Maximizing Treatment Effectiveness: Early detection allows for the timely initiation of appropriate treatments and lifestyle modifications. The earlier treatment begins, the more effective it is in slowing down bone loss and increasing bone density. Delaying treatment can result in further bone deterioration and increased fracture risk.

• Preventing Complications: Osteoporosis-related fractures can lead to a range of complications, including pneumonia, blood clots, pressure sores, and a decline in overall health. Early detection and management can help prevent these complications, reducing the burden on both patients and healthcare systems.

• Improved Quality of Life: Osteoporosis can significantly impact an individual's quality of life due to pain, physical limitations, and the fear of falling. Early detection and appropriate interventions can help individuals maintain their independence, mobility, and overall well-being.

• Cost Savings: Detecting osteoporosis early and implementing preventive measures are cost-effective in the long run. Preventing fractures through early intervention reduces the economic burden on healthcare systems associated with hospitalizations, surgeries, and long-term care.

• Tailored Treatment Plans: Early detection allows healthcare providers to develop personalized treatment plans based on an individual's risk factors, bone density measurements, and overall health. This tailored approach ensures that the chosen interventions align with the patient's specific needs and preferences.

• Enhanced Awareness and Education: Early diagnosis can serve as an opportunity to educate individuals about the importance of bone health and the lifestyle changes needed to maintain strong bones. It promotes awareness about osteoporosis risk factors and encourages proactive measures to prevent the condition.

• Secondary Causes: Osteoporosis can sometimes be a result of underlying medical conditions or medications. Identifying osteoporosis early may lead to the discovery and management of these underlying issues, potentially improving overall health.

In summary, early detection of osteoporosis is essential for preventing fractures, maximizing treatment efficacy, minimizing complications, improving quality of life, reducing healthcare costs, and promoting overall bone health. Regular discussions with healthcare providers, bone density testing when indicated, and adherence to recommended preventive measures are crucial steps in achieving early detection and effective management of osteoporosis.

IMPORTANCE OF BONE HEALTH

Bone health is of paramount importance throughout one's life, and it plays a crucial role in overall well-being. Here are several reasons highlighting the significance of bone health:

• Structural Support: Bones provide the framework for the body, allowing us to stand, move, and perform everyday activities. Healthy bones ensure structural integrity and support for the entire body.

• Protection of Vital Organs: Many of the body's vital organs, such as the brain, heart, and lungs, are protected by bones. For instance, the skull protects the brain, the ribcage shields the heart and lungs, and the spine safeguards the spinal cord.

• Mobility and Functionality: Healthy bones enable mobility and the ability to perform a wide range of physical activities. Strong bones are essential for walking, running, lifting, and maintaining balance.

• Muscle Attachment: Muscles attach to bones through tendons, allowing us to move our limbs and perform various movements. Healthy bones provide a stable anchor for muscles to exert force.

• Mineral Storage: Bones act as a reservoir for essential minerals, primarily calcium and phosphorus. When the body needs these minerals for various functions, such as muscle contraction and nerve signaling, it can draw upon bone stores.

• Blood Cell Production: Bone marrow, found within certain bones, is responsible for the production of blood cells, including red blood cells (which carry oxygen) and white blood cells (which play a role in the immune system). Healthy bone marrow is critical for overall health.

• Endocrine Function: Bones produce hormones that regulate various physiological processes, such as energy metabolism and glucose homeostasis. For example, osteocalcin, a hormone produced by bones, influences insulin sensitivity.

• Balance and Posture: Strong and healthy bones, particularly those in the spine, contribute to good posture and balance. Maintaining proper posture is essential for preventing musculoskeletal pain and injuries.

• Long-Term Health: Building and maintaining strong bones during youth and adulthood is crucial for preventing osteoporosis and fractures later in life. Osteoporosis can lead to serious health consequences, including pain, disability, and a reduced quality of life.

• Quality of Life: Good bone health enhances overall quality of life by allowing individuals to remain active, independent, and free from chronic pain and disability.

• Healthy Aging: As people age, maintaining bone health becomes increasingly important. Strong bones in older age reduce the risk of falls band fractures, contributing to a higher level of independence and a better quality of life.

• Prevention of Chronic Diseases: There is growing evidence suggesting that bone health may be linked to other chronic conditions, including cardiovascular disease and certain cancers. Maintaining healthy bones may have positive effects on overall health.

In conclusion, bone health is fundamental to daily life, mobility, and overall well-being. It plays a vital role in protecting vital organs, providing support for the body, and enabling physical activity. Investing in bone health through proper nutrition, regular exercise, and lifestyle choices is essential for maintaining a high quality of life throughout one's lifespan.

OSTEOPOROSIS DIET

A diet for osteoporosis focuses on increasing bone density and reducing the risk of fractures. Osteoporosis is a condition characterized by weakened bones, so it's important to provide your body with the right nutrients to support bone health. Here's a diet plan and dietary guidelines to consider if you have osteoporosis:

1. Calcium-Rich Foods: Calcium is vital for bone health. Aim to get 1,000 to 1,300 milligrams of calcium per day, depending on your age and gender. Include the following calcium-rich foods in your diet:

• Dairy products: Low-fat or fat-free milk, yogurt, and cheese.

• Fortified plant-based milk: Almond, soy, or oat milk fortified with calcium.

• Leafy green vegetables: Kale, collard greens, broccoli, and bok choy.

• Tofu: Opt for tofu made with calcium sulfate.

• Canned fish: Salmon and sardines with bones are good sources.

2. Vitamin D: Vitamin D is essential for calcium absorption. Spend some time in the sun and consume foods rich in vitamin D:

• Fatty fish: Salmon, mackerel, and trout.

• Fortified dairy or plant-based milk.

• Egg yolks.

• Cod liver oil.

3. Magnesium: Magnesium is important for bone health as it aids in calcium absorption. Include magnesium-rich foods in your diet:

• Nuts and seeds: Almonds, sunflower seeds, and pumpkin seeds.

• Whole grains: Brown rice, quinoa, and whole wheat.

• Leafy green vegetables: Spinach, Swiss chard, and kale.

4. Vitamin K: Vitamin K plays a role in bone mineralization. Consume foods rich in vitamin K:

• Leafy green vegetables: Kale, spinach, and collard greens.

• Brussels sprouts.

• Broccoli.

• Cabbage.

5. Protein: Protein is a key component of bone tissue. Include lean sources of protein in your diet:

• Lean meats: Chicken, turkey, and lean cuts of beef.

• Fish: Salmon, trout, and tuna.

• Legumes: Beans, lentils, and chickpeas.

• Tofu and tempeh.

6. Phosphorus: Phosphorus works alongside calcium to strengthen bones. Consume phosphorus-rich foods:

• Dairy products: Milk, yogurt, and cheese.

• Meat: Chicken, turkey, and lean beef.

• Fish: Salmon, trout, and tuna.

• Nuts and seeds.

7. Limit Sodium and Caffeine: High sodium and caffeine intake can lead to calcium loss in urine. Reduce your consumption of processed foods high in salt and moderate your caffeine intake.

8. Limit Alcohol: Excessive alcohol consumption can weaken bones. If you drink alcohol, do so in moderation.

9. Maintain a Healthy Weight: Being underweight can increase the risk of fractures in individuals with osteoporosis. Aim to maintain a healthy body weight through a balanced diet and regular exercise.

10. Engage in Weight-Bearing Exercise: Incorporate weight-bearing exercises like walking, dancing, and weightlifting into your routine to stimulate bone growth.

11. Consult a Healthcare Provider: If you have osteoporosis, consult with your healthcare provider or a registered dietitian to develop a personalized diet and lifestyle plan that addresses your specific needs and concerns.

Remember that consistency in following a bone-healthy diet, along with lifestyle modifications, can help manage osteoporosis and reduce the risk of fractures. It's important to work with a healthcare professional to create a plan tailored to your individual needs.

Lifestyle changes play a significant and multifaceted role in promoting and maintaining overall health and well-being. They have a profound impact on various aspects of physical, mental, and emotional health, as well as the prevention and management of numerous chronic diseases. Here are several key reasons highlighting the significance of lifestyle changes:

• Prevention of Chronic Diseases: Many chronic diseases, including heart disease, diabetes, obesity, and certain types of cancer, are strongly influenced by lifestyle factors such as diet, physical activity, and tobacco use. Making positive lifestyle changes can significantly reduce the risk of these diseases.

• Improved Cardiovascular Health: Healthy lifestyle choices, such as a balanced diet, regular physical activity, and stress management, contribute to better cardiovascular health. They can help lower blood pressure, reduce cholesterol levels, and decrease the risk of heart disease and stroke.

• Weight Management: Adopting a healthy lifestyle that includes a nutritious diet and regular exercise is crucial for achieving and maintaining a healthy weight. Weight management is linked to a reduced risk of obesity-related conditions and improved overall health.

• Enhanced Mental Health: Lifestyle changes can have a positive impact on mental health by reducing stress, anxiety, and depression. Regular exercise, a balanced diet, and adequate sleep are known to support emotional well-being.

• Improved Quality of Life: Healthy lifestyle choices can enhance overall quality of life by increasing energy levels, improving sleep, and reducing the risk of chronic pain and discomfort. This leads to a greater sense of vitality and well-being.

• Prevention of Osteoporosis: Lifestyle factors such as adequate calcium and vitamin D intake, weight-bearing exercise, and avoiding excessive alcohol and tobacco use are essential for maintaining strong and healthy bones and reducing the risk of osteoporosis.

• Cancer Prevention: Healthy lifestyle changes, such as maintaining a healthy weight, eating a balanced diet rich in fruits and vegetables, and avoiding tobacco and excessive alcohol use, can reduce the risk of certain cancers.

• Enhanced Immune Function: A healthy lifestyle supports a strong immune system, making the body better equipped to defend against infections and illnesses.

• Longevity: A healthy lifestyle is associated with a longer life expectancy. People who make positive lifestyle changes tend to live longer and enjoy a higher quality of life in their later years.

• Reduced Healthcare Costs: By preventing chronic diseases and promoting overall health, lifestyle changes can lead to lower healthcare costs for individuals and society as a whole.

• Positive Role Modeling: Making healthy lifestyle changes can serve as a positive example for family members and friends, encouraging them to make similar choices and improve their health.

• Environmental Impact: Sustainable lifestyle changes, such as reducing waste, conserving energy, and adopting plant-based diets, can have a positive impact on the environment and contribute to a more sustainable future.

In conclusion, lifestyle changes are instrumental in preventing chronic diseases, promoting mental and physical health, enhancing overall well-being, and contributing to a longer, healthier life. The significance of these changes cannot be overstated, as they empower individuals to take control of their health and make choices that lead to a happier and more fulfilling life.

PART TWO

Greek Yogurt Parfait

Ingredients:

• Greek yogurt

• Fresh berries (e.g., strawberries, blueberries)

• Chopped nuts (e.g., almonds, walnuts)

• Honey (optional)

Instructions:

1. Layer Greek yogurt, fresh berries, and chopped nuts in a bowl or glass.

2. Drizzle with honey for sweetness if desired.

Spinach and Mushroom Omelette

Ingredients:

• Eggs

- Fresh spinach

- Sliced mushrooms

- Shredded cheese (e.g., low-fat Swiss)

- Olive oil

Instructions:

1. Sauté mushrooms and spinach in olive oil until wilted.

2. Whisk eggs and pour them into the pan with sautéed veggies.

3. Sprinkle with cheese, cook until set, and fold the omelette in half.

Overnight Oats

Ingredients:

- Rolled oats

- Milk (e.g., almond, soy, or dairy)

- Chia seeds

- Sliced bananas

• Cinnamon (optional)

Instructions:

1. Mix rolled oats, milk, chia seeds, and sliced bananas in a jar or bowl.

2. Refrigerate overnight and top with a sprinkle of cinnamon in the morning.

Avocado Toast

Ingredients:

• Whole-grain bread

• Ripe avocado

• Sliced tomato

• Sprinkle of sesame seeds

Instructions:

1. Toast whole-grain bread.

2. Mash ripe avocado and spread it on the toast.

3. Top with sliced tomatoes and a sprinkle of sesame seeds.

Berry Smoothie

Ingredients:

• Frozen mixed berries (e.g., strawberries, blueberries, raspberries)

• Greek yogurt

• Spinach leaves

• Almond milk

• Honey (optional)

Instructions:

1. Blend frozen berries, Greek yogurt, spinach leaves, and almond milk until smooth.

2. Sweeten with honey if desired.

Salmon and Cream Cheese Bagel

Ingredients:

• Whole-grain bagel

- Smoked salmon

- Low-fat cream cheese

- Sliced cucumber

- Red onion slices

Instructions:

1. Spread cream cheese on a toasted whole-grain bagel.

2. Layer with smoked salmon, cucumber slices, and red onion.

Veggie Breakfast Burrito

Ingredients:

- Whole-grain tortilla

- Scrambled eggs

- Sautéed bell peppers, onions, and spinach

- Salsa (optional)

Instructions:

1. Fill a whole-grain tortilla with scrambled eggs and sautéed vegetables.

2. Add salsa for extra flavor.

Quinoa Breakfast Bowl

Ingredients:

• Cooked quinoa

• Sliced banana

• Chopped nuts (e.g., almonds, pecans)

• Drizzle of honey

Instructions:

1. Combine cooked quinoa, sliced banana, and chopped nuts in a bowl.

2. Drizzle with honey for sweetness.

Cottage Cheese and Fruit Bowl

Ingredients:

• Low-fat cottage cheese

• Sliced peaches or mixed fruit

• Sprinkle of sunflower seeds

Instructions:

1. Top a bowl of low-fat cottage cheese with sliced peaches or mixed fruit.

2. Sprinkle with sunflower seeds for added crunch.

Pumpkin Spice Oatmeal

Ingredients:

• Rolled oats

• Canned pumpkin puree

• Pumpkin pie spice

• Chopped nuts (e.g., pecans)

Instructions:

• Cook rolled oats with canned pumpkin puree and pumpkin pie spice.

• Top with chopped nuts for added flavor and texture.

Quinoa and Berry Breakfast Bowl

Ingredients:

• 1/2 cup cooked quinoa

• Mixed berries (e.g., blueberries, raspberries)

• Greek yogurt

• Chopped almonds

• Honey (optional)

Instructions:

1. Place cooked quinoa in a bowl.

2. Top with mixed berries, a dollop of Greek yogurt, chopped almonds, and a drizzle of honey for sweetness.

Mediterranean Veggie Scramble

Ingredients:

• Eggs

• Chopped spinach

• Chopped tomatoes

• Chopped red bell peppers

• Feta cheese

• Olive oil

Instructions:

1. In a skillet, sauté chopped spinach, tomatoes, and red bell peppers in olive oil until softened.

2. Pour beaten eggs over the veggies and scramble.

3. Top with crumbled feta cheese.

Pumpkin and Chia Seed Porridge

Ingredients:

• Rolled oats

• Canned pumpkin puree

• Chia seeds

• Pumpkin pie spice

• Sliced bananas

Instructions:

1. Cook rolled oats with canned pumpkin puree, chia seeds, and a sprinkle of pumpkin pie spice.

2. Top with sliced bananas.

Salmon and Spinach Breakfast Wrap

Ingredients:

• Whole-grain tortilla

• Smoked salmon

• Sautéed spinach

• Scrambled eggs

• Low-fat cream cheese

Instructions:

1. Spread low-fat cream cheese on a whole-grain tortilla.

2. Layer with smoked salmon, sautéed spinach, and scrambled eggs.

3. Roll up the tortilla into a wrap.

Peach and Walnut Yogurt Parfait

Ingredients:

• Low-fat yogurt

• Sliced peaches (canned or fresh)

• Chopped walnuts

• Ground cinnamon

Instructions:

1. In a glass, layer low-fat yogurt, sliced peaches, and chopped walnuts.

2. Sprinkle with a pinch of ground cinnamon.

Chia Seed Pudding with Almonds and Berries

Ingredients:

• Chia seeds

- Almond milk

- Sliced almonds

- Mixed berries

- Honey (optional)

Instructions:

1. Mix chia seeds and almond milk in a jar, and refrigerate overnight.

2. In the morning, top with sliced almonds, mixed berries, and a drizzle of honey.

Broccoli and Cheese Frittata

Ingredients:

- Eggs

- Chopped broccoli florets

- Shredded low-fat cheese

- Chopped onions

• Olive oil

Instructions:

• Sauté chopped broccoli and onions in olive oil until tender.

• Pour beaten eggs over the veggies, sprinkle with shredded cheese, and cook until set.

Berry and Spinach Smoothie Bowl

Ingredients:

• Frozen mixed berries

• Fresh spinach leaves

• Greek yogurt

• Almond milk

• Ground flaxseed

Instructions:

1. Blend frozen berries, spinach, Greek yogurt, almond milk, and ground flaxseed until smooth.

2. Pour into a bowl and top with additional berries or granola if desired.

Oat Bran Pancakes

Ingredients:

- Oat bran

- Whole-wheat flour

- Baking powder

- Low-fat milk

- Egg whites

Instructions:

1. Mix oat bran, whole-wheat flour, and baking powder in a bowl.

2. Add low-fat milk and egg whites to create a pancake batter.

3. Cook pancakes on a griddle until golden brown.

Tomato and Basil Breakfast Sandwich

Ingredients:

- Whole-grain English muffin

- Sliced tomatoes

- Fresh basil leaves

- Poached or fried egg

- Low-fat mozzarella cheese

Instructions:

1. Toast a whole-grain English muffin.

2. Layer with sliced tomatoes, fresh basil leaves, a poached or fried egg, and low-fat mozzarella cheese.

Greek Yogurt Parfait with Nuts and Berries

Ingredients:

- Greek yogurt

- Mixed berries (e.g., strawberries, blueberries, raspberries)

- Chopped nuts (e.g., almonds, walnuts)

- Honey (optional)

Instructions:

1. In a glass or bowl, layer Greek yogurt, mixed berries, and chopped nuts.

2. Drizzle with honey if desired.

3. Enjoy this calcium and protein-rich parfait.

Spinach and Feta Omelette

Ingredients:

• Eggs

• Chopped spinach

• Crumbled feta cheese

• Chopped tomatoes

• Chopped onions

• Olive oil

Instructions:

1. In a bowl, beat eggs with a pinch of salt and pepper.

2. In a non-stick skillet, sauté chopped spinach, chopped tomatoes, and chopped onions in olive oil until softened.

3. Pour beaten eggs over the vegetables and cook until set.

4. Sprinkle crumbled feta cheese on one half of the omelette, fold it over, and serve.

Oatmeal with Almond Butter and Banana

Ingredients:

• Rolled oats

• Almond butter

• Sliced bananas

• Chopped almonds

• Cinnamon

• Honey (optional)

Instructions:

1. Cook rolled oats with water or milk according to package instructions.

2. Top the oatmeal with almond butter, sliced bananas, chopped almonds, and a sprinkle of cinnamon.

3. Drizzle with honey if desired.

Whole-Grain Pancakes with Blueberries

Ingredients:

• Whole-grain pancake mix

• Fresh or frozen blueberries

• Low-fat yogurt

• Maple syrup (optional)

Instructions:

1. Prepare whole-grain pancake batter according to the package instructions.

2. Add fresh or frozen blueberries to the batter.

3. Cook pancakes on a griddle or skillet until golden brown.

4. Serve with a dollop of low-fat yogurt and a drizzle of maple syrup if desired.

Avocado Toast with Poached Eggs

Ingredients:

• Whole-grain bread

• Ripe avocado

• Eggs

• Lemon juice

• Red pepper flakes (optional)

Instructions:

1. Toast whole-grain bread.

2. Mash ripe avocado with a squeeze of lemon juice and a pinch of red pepper flakes (if desired).

3. Poach eggs to your preferred level of doneness.

4. Spread the mashed avocado on the toast and top with poached eggs.

Spinach and Mushroom Breakfast Quesadilla

Ingredients:

• Whole-grain tortillas

• Sautéed spinach and mushrooms

• Scrambled eggs

• Low-fat cheese (shredded)

Instructions:

1. Lay out whole-grain tortillas.

2. Spread sautéed spinach, mushrooms, scrambled eggs, and shredded low-fat cheese on one half of each tortilla.

3. Fold the tortillas in half and cook on a skillet until they are golden brown and the cheese is melted.

Yogurt and Berry Smoothie Bowl

Ingredients:

• Greek yogurt

• Mixed berries (e.g., strawberries, blueberries, raspberries)

• Chia seeds

• Honey (optional)

Instructions:

1. In a bowl, layer Greek yogurt and mixed berries.

2. Sprinkle with chia seeds and drizzle with honey if desired.

3. Customize with your favorite toppings like chopped nuts or granola.

Tofu Scramble with Broccoli and Red Peppers

Ingredients:

• Firm tofu (crumbled)

• Chopped broccoli

• Sliced red bell peppers

• Chopped onions

• Turmeric (for color)

• Olive oil

Instructions:

1. In a skillet, sauté chopped onions until translucent.

2. Add crumbled tofu, chopped broccoli, and sliced red bell peppers.

3. Season with turmeric for color and cook until the tofu is heated through and the vegetables are tender.

Whole-Grain Waffles with Greek Yogurt and Berries

Ingredients:

• Whole-grain waffles (store-bought or homemade)

• Greek yogurt

• Mixed berries (e.g., blueberries, strawberries)

• Maple syrup (optional)

Instructions:

1. Toast whole-grain waffles until crispy.

2. Top with a generous dollop of Greek yogurt and mixed berries.

3. Drizzle with maple syrup if desired.

Chia Seed Pudding with Almonds and Mango

Ingredients:

• Chia seeds

• Almond milk

• Sliced almonds

• Fresh mango chunks

• Vanilla extract

Instructions:

1. In a bowl, mix chia seeds, almond milk, and a drop of vanilla extract. Stir well and refrigerate overnight or until the mixture thickens.

2. Serve in a glass or bowl, topped with sliced almonds and fresh mango chunks.

Grilled Chicken and Broccoli Quinoa Bowl

Ingredients:

• Grilled chicken breast

• Steamed broccoli florets

• Cooked quinoa

• Sliced cherry tomatoes

• Olive oil

• Lemon juice

• Fresh parsley (optional)

Instructions:

1. Arrange grilled chicken, steamed broccoli, and cooked quinoa in a bowl. Top with sliced cherry tomatoes.

2. Drizzle with a mixture of olive oil and lemon juice. Garnish with fresh parsley if desired.

Salmon Salad with Avocado Dressing

Ingredients:

• Grilled or baked salmon fillet

• Mixed greens (e.g., spinach, arugula)

• Sliced cucumbers

• Sliced red onions

• Avocado

• Greek yogurt

• Lemon juice

• Dill (optional)

Instructions:

1. Combine mixed greens, sliced cucumbers, and red onions in a salad bowl.

2. In a blender, blend avocado, Greek yogurt, lemon juice, and dill until creamy.

3. Drizzle the avocado dressing over the salad and top with grilled or baked salmon.

Ingredients:

• Firm tofu cubes

• Assorted stir-fry vegetables (e.g., bell peppers, broccoli, carrots)

• Low-sodium soy sauce

• Garlic and ginger (minced)

• Sesame oil

• Brown rice

Instructions:

1. In a wok or skillet, stir-fry tofu cubes until golden brown. Remove from the pan.

2. In the same pan, stir-fry the assorted vegetables with minced garlic and ginger until tender.

3. Return tofu to the pan, add low-sodium soy sauce, and drizzle with sesame oil.

4. Serve over cooked brown rice.

Ingredients:

• Bell peppers (any color)

• Sautéed mushrooms

• Sautéed spinach

• Cooked quinoa

• Low-fat mozzarella cheese

• Tomato sauce

Instructions:

1. Cut the tops off the bell peppers and remove seeds and membranes.

2. Stuff the peppers with sautéed mushrooms, sautéed spinach, cooked quinoa, and a sprinkle of low-fat mozzarella cheese.

3. Place the stuffed peppers in a baking dish, pour tomato sauce over them, and bake until peppers are tender.

Chickpea and Vegetable Soup

Ingredients:

• Chickpeas (canned or cooked)

• Assorted vegetables (e.g., carrots, celery, zucchini)

• Low-sodium vegetable broth

• Garlic and onion (minced)

• Italian seasoning

• Spinach leaves

Instructions:

1. In a large pot, sauté minced garlic and onion until fragrant.

2. Add assorted vegetables and cook until slightly softened. Stir in chickpeas, low-sodium vegetable broth, and Italian seasoning.

3. Simmer until vegetables are tender. Add spinach leaves and cook until wilted.

Spinach and Feta Stuffed Chicken Breast

Ingredients:

• Boneless, skinless chicken breasts

• Fresh spinach leaves

• Crumbled feta cheese

• Garlic powder

• Olive oil

• Lemon juice

Instructions:

1. Preheat the oven to 375°F (190°C).

2. Butterfly the chicken breasts and season with garlic powder. Lay a handful of fresh spinach and crumbled feta cheese on each chicken breast.

3. Roll up the chicken breasts and secure with toothpicks. Drizzle with olive oil and lemon juice.

4. Bake for 25-30 minutes or until the chicken is cooked through.

Quinoa and Black Bean Salad

Ingredients:

• Cooked quinoa

• Black beans (canned, rinsed, and drained)

• Chopped bell peppers (various colors)

• Chopped red onion

• Fresh cilantro leaves

• Lime vinaigrette (lime juice, olive oil, honey)

Instructions:

1. In a large bowl, combine cooked quinoa, black beans, chopped bell peppers, chopped red onion, and fresh cilantro.

2. Drizzle with lime vinaigrette and toss to combine.

3. Serve as a cold salad.

Tuna and White Bean Salad

Ingredients:

• Canned tuna (in water, drained)

• Canned white beans (cannellini or navy, drained and rinsed)

• Chopped celery

• Chopped red onion

• Dijon mustard

• Olive oil

• Lemon juice

Instructions:

1. In a bowl, combine canned tuna, white beans, chopped celery, and chopped red onion.

2. In a separate bowl, whisk together Dijon mustard, olive oil, and lemon juice to make a dressing.

3. Drizzle the dressing over the salad and toss to coat.

Sweet Potato and Lentil Soup

Ingredients:

• Sweet potatoes (peeled and diced)

• Red lentils

• Chopped carrots

• Chopped celery

• Vegetable broth

• Ground cumin

• Paprika

• Salt and pepper

Instructions:

1. In a large pot, combine sweet potatoes, red lentils, chopped carrots, and chopped celery.

2. Add vegetable broth, ground cumin, paprika, salt, and pepper.

3. Simmer until the vegetables and lentils are soft.

4. Blend the soup until smooth.

Greek Chickpea Salad

Ingredients:

• Canned chickpeas (drained and rinsed)

• Cherry tomatoes (halved)

• Cucumber (diced)

• Red onion (thinly sliced)

• Kalamata olives (pitted and sliced)

• Feta cheese (crumbled)

• Greek dressing (olive oil, lemon juice, garlic, oregano)

Instructions:

1. In a large bowl, combine chickpeas, cherry tomatoes, cucumber, red onion, Kalamata olives, and crumbled feta cheese.

2. In a separate bowl, whisk together Greek dressing ingredients.

3. Drizzle the dressing over the salad and toss to combine.

Salmon and Asparagus Quiche

Ingredients:

• Pie crust (whole-grain, if available)

• Salmon fillets

• Fresh asparagus spears

• Eggs

• Low-fat milk

• Shredded Swiss cheese

• Dill (fresh or dried)

Instructions:

1. Preheat the oven to 375°F (190°C). Bake the pie crust until lightly golden.

2. In a separate pan, cook salmon and asparagus until tender. In a bowl, whisk eggs, low-fat milk, shredded Swiss cheese, and dill.

3. Arrange the cooked salmon and asparagus in the pie crust and pour the egg mixture over them. Bake for about 30 minutes or until the quiche is set and golden.

Veggie and Chickpea Stir-Fry

Ingredients:

• Chickpeas (canned, drained and rinsed)

• Sliced bell peppers (various colors)

• Sliced carrots

• Broccoli florets

• Snap peas

• Low-sodium soy sauce

• Garlic and ginger (minced)

• Brown rice

Instructions:

1. In a wok or skillet, stir-fry chickpeas, sliced bell peppers, carrots, broccoli, and snap peas with minced garlic and ginger.

2. Add a splash of low-sodium soy sauce for flavor.

3. Serve the stir-fry over cooked brown rice.

Mushroom and Spinach Stuffed Whole-Grain Pita

Ingredients:

• Whole-grain pita bread

• Sautéed mushrooms

• Sautéed spinach

• Hummus

• Sliced tomatoes

Instructions:

1. Warm the whole-grain pita bread.

2. Stuff the pita with sautéed mushrooms, sautéed spinach, a generous spread of hummus, and sliced tomatoes.

Ingredients:

• Green or brown lentils

• Chopped carrots

• Chopped celery

• Chopped onions

• Low-sodium vegetable broth

• Crushed tomatoes

• Fresh thyme leaves

• Salt and pepper

Instructions:

1. In a large pot, combine lentils, chopped carrots, chopped celery, chopped onions, low-sodium vegetable broth, crushed tomatoes, fresh thyme leaves, salt, and pepper.

2. Simmer until the lentils and vegetables are tender.

Avocado and Black Bean Salad

Ingredients:

- Ripe avocados

- Canned black beans (drained and rinsed)

- Corn kernels (fresh or frozen)

- Chopped red onions

- Chopped cilantro

- Lime juice

- Olive oil

Instructions:

1. In a bowl, combine ripe avocados, black beans, corn kernels, chopped red onions, and chopped cilantro.

2. Drizzle with lime juice and olive oil, and gently toss to combine.

Ingredients:

• Cooked quinoa

• Chopped kale

• Sliced oranges or grapefruit

• Chopped almonds

• Feta cheese (optional)

Citrus Vinaigrette:

• Orange or grapefruit juice

• Olive oil

• Dijon mustard

• Honey

Instructions:

1. In a large bowl, combine cooked quinoa, chopped kale, sliced citrus fruit, and chopped almonds.

2. In a separate bowl, whisk together the citrus vinaigrette ingredients.

3. Drizzle the vinaigrette over the salad and toss to coat. Add feta cheese if desired.

Baked Sweet Potato with Chickpea and Spinach Topping

Ingredients:

• Sweet potatoes

• Canned chickpeas (drained and rinsed)

• Chopped spinach

• Chopped red onion

• Olive oil

• Paprika

• Cumin

Instructions:

• Preheat the oven to 400°F (200°C).

• Pierce sweet potatoes with a fork and bake until tender.

• In a pan, sauté chopped red onion, canned chickpeas, chopped spinach, olive oil, paprika, and cumin until spinach is wilted.

• Split the baked sweet potatoes and top with the chickpea and spinach mixture.

Turkey and Avocado Wrap

Ingredients:

• Whole-grain wrap or tortilla

• Sliced turkey breast

• Sliced avocado

• Baby spinach leaves

• Dijon mustard (optional)

Instructions:

1. Lay a whole-grain wrap or tortilla flat.

2. Layer with sliced turkey breast, sliced avocado, baby spinach leaves, and a drizzle of Dijon mustard if desired.

3. Roll up the wrap and cut in half.

Sesame Kale and Tofu Salad

Ingredients:

• Chopped kale

• Baked or pan-fried tofu cubes

• Sliced cucumber

• Shredded carrots

• Sesame seeds

Sesame Ginger Dressing:

• Rice vinegar

• Sesame oil

• Soy sauce (low-sodium)

• Fresh ginger (grated)

• Honey

Instructions:

1. In a large bowl, combine chopped kale, baked or pan-fried tofu cubes, sliced cucumber, and shredded carrots.

2. In a separate bowl, whisk together the sesame ginger dressing ingredients.

3. Drizzle the dressing over the salad, sprinkle with sesame seeds, and toss to combine.

Mediterranean Lentil Soup

Ingredients:

• Green or brown lentils

• Chopped onions

• Chopped carrots

• Chopped celery

• Minced garlic

• Vegetable broth (low-sodium)

- Chopped tomatoes

- Ground cumin

- Paprika

- Fresh parsley (chopped)

Instructions:

- In a large pot, combine green or brown lentils, chopped onions, chopped carrots, chopped celery, minced garlic, vegetable broth, chopped tomatoes, ground cumin, and paprika.

- Simmer until lentils and vegetables are tender.

- Serve garnished with fresh parsley.

Mushroom and Spinach Quinoa Bowl

Ingredients:

- Cooked quinoa

- Sautéed mushrooms

- Sautéed spinach

• Chopped roasted red peppers

• Feta cheese (optional)

Instructions:

1. Layer cooked quinoa, sautéed mushrooms, sautéed spinach, and chopped roasted red peppers in a bowl.

2. Sprinkle with feta cheese if desired.

Black Bean and Vegetable Quesadilla

Ingredients:

• Whole-grain tortilla

• Black beans (canned, rinsed, and mashed)

• Sliced bell peppers

• Sliced red onions

• Shredded low-fat cheese

• Salsa (optional)

Instructions:

1. Spread mashed black beans on a whole-grain tortilla.

2. Top with sliced bell peppers, sliced red onions, and shredded low-fat cheese.

3. Fold in half and cook on a skillet until cheese is melted.

4. Serve with salsa if desired.

Chickpea and Avocado Salad

Ingredients:

• Canned chickpeas (drained and rinsed)

• Diced avocado

• Chopped cucumber

• Chopped red onion

• Chopped cilantro

• Lime juice

• Olive oil

Instructions:

1. In a bowl, combine canned chickpeas, diced avocado, chopped cucumber, chopped red onion, and chopped cilantro.

2. Drizzle with lime juice and olive oil, and gently toss to combine.

Lentil and Spinach Stuffed Bell Peppers

Ingredients:

• Bell peppers (any color)

• Cooked green or brown lentils

• Sautéed spinach

• Chopped tomatoes

• Shredded low-fat cheese

Instructions:

1. Cut the tops off bell peppers and remove seeds and membranes.

2. Stuff the peppers with cooked lentils, sautéed spinach, chopped tomatoes, and shredded low-fat cheese.

3. Place the stuffed peppers in a baking dish and bake until peppers are tender.

Ingredients:

• Cooked chicken breast (shredded)

• Cooked quinoa

• Chopped carrots

• Chopped celery

• Chopped onions

• Low-sodium chicken broth

• Fresh thyme leaves

Instructions:

1. In a pot, combine shredded cooked chicken breast, cooked quinoa, chopped carrots, chopped celery, chopped onions, low-sodium chicken broth, and fresh thyme leaves.

2. Simmer until vegetables are tender.

Ingredients:

- Whole-grain wrap or tortilla

- Scrambled eggs

- Sliced tomatoes

- Sliced bell peppers

- Sliced avocado

Instructions:

- Lay a whole-grain wrap or tortilla flat.

- Fill with scrambled eggs, sliced tomatoes, sliced bell peppers, and sliced avocado.

- Roll up the wrap and enjoy.

Tuna and Quinoa Salad

Ingredients:

- Canned tuna (in water, drained)

- Cooked quinoa

- Sliced cucumbers

- Cherry tomatoes (halved)

- Kalamata olives (pitted and sliced)

- Greek dressing (olive oil, lemon juice, oregano)

Instructions:

1. In a bowl, combine canned tuna, cooked quinoa, sliced cucumbers, cherry tomatoes, and Kalamata olives.

2. Drizzle with Greek dressing and toss to combine.

Veggie and Hummus Wrap

Ingredients:

- Whole-grain wrap or tortilla

- Hummus

- Sliced cucumbers

- Sliced bell peppers

• Sliced red onions

• Baby spinach leaves

Instructions:

• Lay a whole-grain wrap or tortilla flat.

• Spread hummus over the wrap and layer with sliced cucumbers, sliced bell peppers, sliced red onions, and baby spinach leaves.

• Roll up the wrap and enjoy.

Tomato and Basil Quinoa Salad

Ingredients:

• Cooked quinoa

• Chopped tomatoes

• Fresh basil leaves

• Balsamic vinaigrette (balsamic vinegar, olive oil, Dijon mustard)

Instructions:

• In a bowl, combine cooked quinoa, chopped tomatoes, and fresh basil leaves.

• Drizzle with balsamic vinaigrette and toss to combine.

Turkey and Cranberry Wrap

Ingredients:

• Whole-grain wrap or tortilla

• Sliced turkey breast

• Fresh spinach leaves

• Cranberry sauce (low-sugar)

• Chopped pecans

Instructions:

1. Lay a whole-grain wrap or tortilla flat.

2. Layer with sliced turkey breast, fresh spinach leaves, cranberry sauce, and chopped pecans.

3. Roll up the wrap and enjoy.

Salmon and Quinoa Stuffed Peppers

Ingredients:

• Bell peppers (any color)

• Baked or grilled salmon

• Cooked quinoa

• Chopped spinach

• Chopped tomatoes

• Olive oil

• Lemon juice

Instructions:

1. Cut the tops off bell peppers and remove seeds and membranes.

2. Fill the peppers with a mixture of baked or grilled salmon, cooked quinoa, chopped spinach, and chopped tomatoes.

3. Drizzle with olive oil and lemon juice.

4. Bake until the peppers are tender.

Vegetable and Chickpea Curry

Ingredients:

• Canned chickpeas (drained and rinsed)

• Mixed vegetables (e.g., cauliflower, carrots, peas)

• Chopped onions

• Coconut milk

• Curry powder

• Garlic and ginger (minced)

• Olive oil

Instructions:

1. In a large pan, sauté minced garlic and minced ginger in olive oil until fragrant.

2. Add chopped onions and mixed vegetables. Cook until softened.

3. Stir in canned chickpeas, coconut milk, and curry powder.

4. Simmer until the vegetables are tender.

Baked Sweet Potato and Black Bean Quesadillas

Ingredients:

• Whole-grain tortillas

• Mashed sweet potatoes

• Canned black beans (drained and rinsed)

• Sliced bell peppers

• Sliced red onions

• Low-fat cheese (shredded)

Instructions:

1. Lay out whole-grain tortillas.

2. Spread mashed sweet potatoes on half of each tortilla.

3. Top with black beans, sliced bell peppers, sliced red onions, and shredded low-fat cheese.

4. Fold the tortillas in half and cook on a skillet until golden brown.

Mushroom and Spinach Risotto

Ingredients:

• Arborio rice

• Sliced mushrooms

• Chopped spinach

• Chopped onions

• Low-sodium vegetable broth

• White wine (optional)

• Parmesan cheese (grated)

Instructions:

1. In a large skillet, sauté chopped onions and sliced mushrooms until soft.

2. Add Arborio rice and cook for a few minutes.

3. Pour in white wine (if using) and cook until it's mostly absorbed.

4. Gradually add low-sodium vegetable broth, stirring constantly until the rice is creamy.

5. Stir in chopped spinach and grated Parmesan cheese.

Turkey and Veggie Stir-Fry with Brown Rice

Ingredients:

• Ground turkey

• Sliced bell peppers

• Sliced carrots

• Sliced snow peas

• Low-sodium stir-fry sauce

• Garlic and ginger (minced)

• Brown rice

Instructions:

1. In a wok or skillet, cook ground turkey until browned.

2. Add sliced bell peppers, sliced carrots, and sliced snow peas. Stir-fry until the vegetables are tender.

3. Drizzle with low-sodium stir-fry sauce and serve over cooked brown rice.

Chickpea and Spinach Curry

Ingredients:

• Canned chickpeas (drained and rinsed)

• Chopped spinach

• Chopped onions

• Chopped tomatoes

• Coconut milk

• Curry powder

• Garlic and ginger (minced)

• Olive oil

Instructions:

1. In a large pan, sauté chopped onions, minced garlic, and minced ginger in olive oil until fragrant.

2. Add chopped tomatoes and cook until softened.

3. Stir in canned chickpeas, chopped spinach, coconut milk, and curry powder.

4. Simmer until spinach is wilted and the curry is heated through.

Baked Chicken and Broccoli Casserole

Ingredients:

• Boneless, skinless chicken breasts

• Steamed broccoli florets

• Brown rice

• Low-sodium chicken broth

• Shredded low-fat cheese

• Garlic powder

Instructions:

1. Preheat the oven to 375°F (190°C).

2. In a baking dish, layer cooked brown rice, steamed broccoli florets, and boneless, skinless chicken breasts.

3. Sprinkle with garlic powder and pour low-sodium chicken broth over the casserole.

4. Top with shredded low-fat cheese and bake until the chicken is cooked through.

Lentil and Sweet Potato Stew

Ingredients:

• Brown or green lentils

• Chopped sweet potatoes

• Chopped carrots

• Chopped celery

• Chopped onions

• Low-sodium vegetable broth

- Ground cumin

- Paprika

Instructions:

1. In a large pot, combine brown or green lentils, chopped sweet potatoes, chopped carrots, chopped celery, chopped onions, low-sodium vegetable broth, ground cumin, and paprika.

2. Simmer until lentils and vegetables are tender.

Shrimp and Spinach Fettuccine Alfredo

Ingredients:

- Whole-grain fettuccine pasta

- Shrimp (peeled and deveined)

- Chopped spinach

- Low-fat cream cheese

- Parmesan cheese (grated)

- Garlic powder

• Olive oil

Instructions:

1. Cook whole-grain fettuccine pasta according to package instructions.

2. In a pan, sauté shrimp in olive oil until cooked.

3. Add chopped spinach, low-fat cream cheese, grated Parmesan cheese, and garlic powder.

4. Stir until the sauce is creamy and the spinach is wilted.

5. Serve the shrimp and spinach Alfredo over cooked fettuccine.

Beef and Broccoli Stir-Fry

Ingredients:

• Lean beef strips

• Broccoli florets

• Sliced bell peppers

• Sliced carrots

• Low-sodium soy sauce

• Garlic and ginger (minced)

• Brown rice

Instructions:

1. In a wok or skillet, stir-fry lean beef strips until browned.

2. Add sliced bell peppers, sliced carrots, minced garlic, and minced ginger. Continue to stir-fry until vegetables are tender.

3. Drizzle with low-sodium soy sauce and serve over cooked brown rice.

Baked Eggplant Parmesan

Ingredients:

• Sliced eggplant

• Whole-wheat breadcrumbs

• Egg whites

• Marinara sauce (low-sodium)

- Part-skim mozzarella cheese (shredded)

- Fresh basil leaves

Instructions:

1. Preheat the oven to 375°F (190°C).

2. Dip eggplant slices in egg whites, then coat with whole-wheat breadcrumbs.

3. Arrange the coated eggplant slices in a baking dish, layer with marinara sauce, and sprinkle with shredded mozzarella cheese.

4. Bake until the eggplant is tender and the cheese is melted and bubbly.

5. Garnish with fresh basil leaves.

Vegetable and Lentil Curry

Ingredients:

- Brown or green lentils

- Chopped cauliflower

- Chopped bell peppers

- Chopped tomatoes

- Coconut milk

- Curry powder

- Garlic and ginger (minced)

- Olive oil

Instructions:

1. In a large pan, sauté minced garlic and minced ginger in olive oil until fragrant.

2. Add chopped cauliflower, chopped bell peppers, and chopped tomatoes. Cook until softened.

3. Stir in cooked brown or green lentils, coconut milk, and curry powder.

4. Simmer until the vegetables are tender.

Mediterranean Grilled Chicken Salad

Ingredients:

• Grilled chicken breast

• Mixed greens (e.g., Romaine, arugula)

• Cherry tomatoes

• Cucumber slices

• Kalamata olives (pitted)

• Feta cheese (crumbled)

• Greek dressing (olive oil, lemon juice, oregano)

Instructions:

1. Arrange grilled chicken breast on a bed of mixed greens.

2. Top with cherry tomatoes, cucumber slices, Kalamata olives, and crumbled feta cheese.

3. Drizzle with Greek dressing and serve.

Vegetable and Tofu Stir-Fry with Brown Rice

Ingredients:

• Firm tofu cubes

• Assorted stir-fry vegetables (e.g., broccoli, snow peas, bell peppers)

• Low-sodium stir-fry sauce

• Garlic and ginger (minced)

• Brown rice

Instructions:

1. In a wok or skillet, stir-fry firm tofu cubes until golden brown. Remove from the pan.

2. Stir-fry assorted vegetables, minced garlic, and minced ginger until tender.

3. Return tofu to the pan, add low-sodium stir-fry sauce, and stir until heated through.

4. Serve over cooked brown rice.

Baked Cod with Spinach and Tomatoes

Ingredients:

• Cod fillets

• Baby spinach leaves

• Cherry tomatoes (halved)

• Garlic (minced)

• Olive oil

• Lemon juice

Instructions:

1. Preheat the oven to 375°F (190°C).

2. Season cod fillets with minced garlic, olive oil, and lemon juice.

3. Place the fillets on a baking sheet and surround them with baby spinach leaves and halved cherry tomatoes.

4. Bake until the cod is cooked through and flakes easily.

Chickpea and Vegetable Curry

Ingredients:

• Canned chickpeas (drained and rinsed)

- Chopped zucchini

- Chopped bell peppers

- Chopped onions

- Coconut milk

- Curry powder

- Garlic and ginger (minced)

- Basmati rice

Instructions:

1. In a large pan, sauté minced garlic and minced ginger until fragrant.

2. Add chopped zucchini, chopped bell peppers, and chopped onions. Cook until softened.

3. Stir in canned chickpeas, coconut milk, and curry powder.

4. Simmer until the vegetables are tender.

5. Serve over cooked Basmati rice.

Turkey and Quinoa Stuffed Acorn Squash

Ingredients:

• Acorn squash (halved and seeded)

• Ground turkey

• Cooked quinoa

• Chopped kale

• Chopped apples

• Cinnamon

Instructions:

1. Preheat the oven to 375°F (190°C).

2. Place acorn squash halves, cut side down, on a baking sheet. Roast until tender.

3. In a pan, cook ground turkey until browned.

4. Mix cooked quinoa, chopped kale, chopped apples, and a pinch of cinnamon into the turkey.

5. Stuff the roasted acorn squash halves with the turkey and quinoa mixture.

Spinach and Mushroom Stuffed Chicken Breast

Ingredients:

• Boneless, skinless chicken breasts

• Sautéed spinach and mushrooms

• Low-fat cream cheese

• Garlic powder

• Olive oil

Instructions:

1. Preheat the oven to 375°F (190°C).

2. Butterfly chicken breasts and season with garlic powder.

3. Spread low-fat cream cheese over each breast and top with sautéed spinach and mushrooms.

4. Fold the chicken breasts over the filling and secure with toothpicks.

5. Bake until the chicken is cooked through.

Ingredients:

- Cooked green or brown lentils

- Mashed sweet potatoes

- Sautéed mixed vegetables (e.g., peas, carrots, corn)

- Low-sodium vegetable broth

- Olive oil

Instructions:

1. In a baking dish, layer cooked lentils and sautéed mixed vegetables.

2. Pour a small amount of low-sodium vegetable broth over the mixture.

3. Spread mashed sweet potatoes on top.

4. Bake until the top is golden and the filling is heated through.

Salmon and Asparagus Foil Packets

Ingredients:

• Salmon fillets

• Asparagus spears

• Sliced lemon

• Fresh dill (optional)

• Olive oil

• Garlic powder

Instructions:

1. Preheat the oven to 375°F (190°C).

2. Place salmon fillets on individual sheets of aluminum foil. Arrange asparagus spears and lemon slices around the salmon.

3. Drizzle with olive oil, sprinkle with garlic powder, and add fresh dill if desired.

4. Seal the foil packets and bake for about 20-25 minutes or until the salmon is cooked through.

Ingredients:

• Cooked quinoa

• Mixed stir-fry vegetables (e.g., broccoli, bell peppers, snap peas)

• Firm tofu cubes (optional)

• Low-sodium soy sauce

• Ginger and garlic (minced)

• Sesame oil

Instructions:

1. In a wok or skillet, stir-fry mixed vegetables and tofu cubes (if using) until tender.

2. Add minced ginger and garlic and continue to cook for a minute.

3. Add cooked quinoa and a drizzle of low-sodium soy sauce and sesame oil. Stir to combine and heat through.

Ingredients:

• Sweet potatoes (cooked and mashed)

• Canned black beans (drained and rinsed)

• Sliced bell peppers

• Chopped onions

• Whole-grain tortillas

• Enchilada sauce (low-sodium)

• Shredded low-fat cheese

Instructions:

1. Preheat the oven to 375°F (190°C).

2. In a bowl, mix mashed sweet potatoes, black beans, sliced bell peppers, and chopped onions.

3. Fill whole-grain tortillas with the mixture and roll them up.

4. Place the rolled enchiladas in a baking dish, cover with low-sodium enchilada sauce, and sprinkle with shredded low-fat cheese.

5. Bake until the cheese is melted and bubbly.

Mushroom and Spinach Stuffed Portobello Mushrooms

Ingredients:

• Portobello mushroom caps

• Sautéed mushrooms and spinach

• Feta cheese (optional)

• Olive oil

• Balsamic vinegar

Instructions:

1. Preheat the oven to 375°F (190°C).

2. Brush Portobello mushroom caps with olive oil and balsamic vinegar.

3. Fill each cap with sautéed mushrooms and spinach, and top with crumbled feta cheese if desired.

4. Bake until the mushrooms are tender and the filling is heated through.

Lentil and Vegetable Tacos

Ingredients:

• Cooked brown or green lentils

• Sliced bell peppers

• Sliced onions

• Sliced avocado

• Whole-grain taco shells

• Salsa (low-sodium)

• Cumin and chili powder

Instructions:

1. In a pan, sauté sliced bell peppers and onions with cumin and chili powder until tender.

2. Warm the whole-grain taco shells in the oven.

3. Fill the taco shells with cooked lentils, sautéed vegetables, sliced avocado, and a dollop of low-sodium salsa.

Lemon Garlic Shrimp and Asparagus Skewers

Ingredients:

• Shrimp (peeled and deveined)

• Asparagus spears

• Lemon juice

• Garlic (minced)

• Olive oil

• Fresh parsley (chopped)

Instructions:

1. In a bowl, combine lemon juice, minced garlic, olive oil, and chopped fresh parsley.

2. Thread shrimp and asparagus onto skewers.

3. Brush the skewers with the lemon garlic mixture.

4. Grill or broil the skewers until the shrimp are pink and cooked through.

Baked Chicken and Broccoli Alfredo

Ingredients:

• Boneless, skinless chicken breasts

• Broccoli florets

• Whole-grain pasta

• Low-fat Alfredo sauce

• Parmesan cheese (grated)

Instructions:

1. Season chicken breasts with your preferred spices and bake until cooked through.

2. Steam broccoli florets until tender.

3. Cook whole-grain pasta according to package instructions.

4. In a saucepan, heat low-fat Alfredo sauce.

5. Slice the cooked chicken and combine it with the steamed broccoli and cooked pasta.

6. Pour the Alfredo sauce over the mixture, sprinkle with grated Parmesan cheese, and bake until bubbly.

Spinach and White Bean Stuffed Bell Peppers

Ingredients:

• Bell peppers (any color)

• Sautéed spinach and white beans

• Low-sodium vegetable broth

• Brown rice

• Parmesan cheese (grated)

Instructions:

1. Cut the tops off bell peppers and remove seeds and membranes.

2. Fill the peppers with a mixture of sautéed spinach and white beans.

3. Place the stuffed peppers in a baking dish, pour low-sodium vegetable broth around them, and bake until peppers are tender.

4. Serve over cooked brown rice and sprinkle with grated Parmesan cheese.

Tofu and Broccoli Stir-Fry

Ingredients:

• Firm tofu cubes

• Broccoli florets

• Sliced bell peppers

• Sliced carrots

• Low-sodium stir-fry sauce

• Garlic and ginger (minced)

• Brown rice

Instructions:

1. In a wok or skillet, stir-fry firm tofu cubes until golden brown.

2. Add broccoli florets, sliced bell peppers, and sliced carrots. Continue to stir-fry until vegetables are tender.

3. Drizzle with low-sodium stir-fry sauce and serve over cooked brown rice.

Mushroom and Spinach Stuffed Chicken Thighs

Ingredients:

• Boneless, skinless chicken thighs

• Sautéed mushrooms and spinach

• Low-fat cream cheese

• Olive oil

• Paprika

Instructions:

1. Preheat the oven to 375°F (190°C).

2. Pound chicken thighs to even thickness.

3. Spread a mixture of sautéed mushrooms and spinach, along with low-fat cream cheese, on each chicken thigh.

4. Roll up the chicken thighs, secure with toothpicks, and brush with olive oil.

5. Sprinkle with paprika and bake until the chicken is cooked through.

CONCLUSION

In conclusion, osteoporosis is a serious medical condition characterized by the weakening of bones, which makes them more susceptible to fractures and breaks. It is often considered a "silent disease" because it progresses without noticeable symptoms until a fracture occurs. However, osteoporosis is preventable and manageable through various dietary and lifestyle strategies.

A comprehensive approach to managing osteoporosis involves not only medical treatment but also a bone-healthy diet that focuses on specific nutrients and foods. Calcium is an essential mineral for maintaining bone health. It's crucial to include calcium-rich foods like dairy products, leafy greens, fortified foods, and supplements if necessary to meet daily calcium requirements. Vitamin D plays a crucial role in calcium absorption. Sun exposure, fortified foods, and supplements can help ensure you have sufficient vitamin D levels. Protein is necessary for bone development and repair. Incorporating lean sources of protein, such as poultry, fish, beans, and tofu, is important for bone health. Vitamin K is involved in bone metabolism. Foods like leafy greens, broccoli, and Brussels sprouts are good sources of vitamin K. Magnesium contributes to bone health and can be found in nuts, seeds, whole grains, and leafy greens. Phosphorus works with calcium to build and maintain strong bones. It is abundant in dairy products, meat, and poultry.

A diet rich in fruits and vegetables provides essential vitamins, minerals, and antioxidants that support overall health and bone density. Excessive sodium and caffeine intake can lead to calcium loss from bones. Reducing the consumption of salty and caffeinated foods and beverages can help preserve bone health. Excessive alcohol consumption can negatively impact bone health. It's advisable to consume alcohol in moderation. Weight-bearing and resistance exercises are essential for strengthening bones and muscles, reducing the risk of falls and fractures. Smoking is associated with lower bone density. Quitting smoking can benefit bone health. Regular bone density tests, especially for individuals at higher risk, can help monitor bone health and guide treatment decisions.

Remember that diet alone cannot completely prevent or treat osteoporosis. It should be combined with other healthy lifestyle choices and, if necessary, medical treatments prescribed by healthcare professionals. Osteoporosis is a condition that can be managed with the right strategies, and a bone-healthy diet plays a significant role in maintaining strong and healthy bones throughout life.